# *You Need Care, Too*

## Table of Contents

| | |
|---|---|
| Forward | 2 |
| Why This Job? | 3 |
| What are Your Beliefs? | 4 |
| Unrealized Grief | 5 |
| Keeping Your Balance | 7 |
| Laughter and Tears | 8 |
| We Can't Fix Everything | 10 |
| We Don't Have to Have All the Answers | 11 |
| We Can't Carry the Pain | 12 |
| Don't Take Negative Behavior Personally | 13 |
| Find Someone to Talk To | 14 |
| Life's Appreciation | 16 |
| Poem | 18 |
| Summary | 19 |

Caring for someone at the end of their life is different than caring for someone who is going to get better. Most people don't know this, even professionals. As a caregiver (nurses, nurse's aides, chaplains, social workers, hired home caregivers, physicians, end of life doulas, eleventh hour and transition volunteers, anyone who is trained to care for a person facing the end of their life) the information in this booklet will give you ideas for taking care of yourself. This is not about how to provide care for others. You know how to do that. This is about caring for you.

Why do you need to take care of yourself? Because working with end of life is not like most of the work we have been trained to do. We are trained to help people get better, not to die. There is something within us that is uncomfortable with - or even rejects - the idea that the end result of our care will be the death of the patient. Add to that our own fears, misconceptions, and often lack of experience with dying and death, and we have a good recipe for burnout.

We also have our peers looking at our role as somehow negative. "How can you work with death all the time? It has to be so depressing." All of this consciously and unconsciously adds stress to our work.

In this booklet I hope to give you some personal tools for staying emotionally healthy so you can continue to do the very special work of helping someone through their final act of living.

# *Why This Job?*

Everything we do we do because it meets a need within ourselves. We tend to think we reach out to others, that we help others, because we are doing it for them. Really we are helping ourselves. It is important to know what draws you to working with people who are dying. Is it because you were in the right place at the right time to get a job, or is it a position you chose? If it's just a job, then it is important to make sure you are comfortable working in this field. If you aren't, get out. Save yourself the pain and frustration.

If you have chosen to work with dying people --why? What has brought you to this unusual work? Is it religious conviction? If so, this is not the work for you. The death bed is not a place to change people's ideology. If it is because you have experienced the death of someone close to you recently, were helped by hospice, and now want to work for them--wait at least a year so that every death doesn't reopen the wound of your own grief. If it is because you are frustrated with how the medical profession is addressing the end of life--welcome! You will feel rewarded. You can make a difference.

## *What Are Your Beliefs?*

A teacher of mine said that we humans are like coffee pots. The clear water we pour into the pot is what happens to us. The coffee grounds are each individual's experiences, beliefs, fears, and memories: our accumulated life. The coffee (water having gone through the coffee grounds) is how we feel about what is happening to us. In other words, how we view the world is distorted by our own experiences and feelings.

A lot of us have scary notions about what it is like to die. In our culture people die out of sight, generally in hospitals and nursing facilities. We tend to avoid the subject of death, as well as physical contact with the dying. If your job requires you to be involved with someone who is dying, you need to stay mentally and emotionally healthy by looking at your own uncomfortable feelings about death.

What are your coffee grounds? What was your first experience with dying and/or death? How old were you? What were your family's ideas regarding death, what were their traditions, what is their culture?

My mother was terrified of death because she accidentally killed a kitten with a rocking chair when she was a child. She passed that fear on to me. It was part of my "coffee grounds" until I looked at it and decided it was unfounded. My fear of driving on bridges and through tunnels was also eliminated at that time of introspection. I haven't done so well with bugs and water. Once you acknowledge those unthought about experiences, and where they came from, you are consciously aware of them. Now you won't carry them from patient to patient. And you won't bring them home as discontent and uneasiness with your work.

## *Unrealized Grief*

You will grieve the loss of your patient whether you know it or not. You have given them a piece of yourself. And having cared for them, you will grieve. The question is how much. Some will touch you more than others. Some will remind you of people in your personal life, some will even fill blank spaces in your life. All will affect you, whether you are aware of it or not.

Most of us go about our job professionally, not

realizing the personal affect that patients have on us. We are competent, do our job, our patient dies, we move on to the next patient, that patient dies and on and on and on. This unconscious accumulation of deaths affects us, but we are unaware of it. We tend to think the relationships we form with our patients are not personal, they are job related, so when our patient dies there is no loss for us. BUT THERE IS. We need to find some way of consciously recognizing those deaths. Then we can release and move on.

I have found that creating a closure ritual is very helpful in dealing with the unrealized grief following the death of a patient. I would go to the visitation as a way of saying goodbye to the body and the family; that was my ritual. I didn't get paid, it was on my own time, but it was good for me. It was my closure.

A helpful tool: create your own ritual. Maybe it is buying a single rose and putting it in a special place in your home. Maybe it is creating a journal with the names of your patients and a blessing. Do whatever you feel is a meaningful way of acknowledging the end of your relationship.

## *Keeping Your Balance*

All work and no play not only makes Jack a dull boy, it also burns him out. We know the right way to live a balanced life. We teach our patients and families what they need to do to stay healthy, but do we practice what we preach? Generally not.

I am not going to go into detail on how to stay healthy. We know what to do, we just don't necessarily do it. We operate under the "do as I say, not do as I do" principle. It is important to consciously act against this tendency. It is easy to do that which is destructive and bad for us and much more difficult to do that which is constructive and good for us. We have to keep our own house in order so that we will have the energy and attention to help others. When our own life is in turmoil it can't help but affect our interactions with others, our patience, our attention, and our stamina.

Areas to try to keep in balance: food, sleep, play, family, and work. A lot of us sacrifice sleep and play for work while overcompensating in the eating department.

Our own families all too often get lost in the shuffle of our busy schedules. They are left to fend for themselves. Often, even when we are at home, we are doing paperwork or thinking about a particular patient or family situation. It is an ongoing challenge to leave work and be fully engaged at home.

In our work environment we offer support, patience, and tenderness all day long. We come home tired, wanting to just go to bed. But we are faced with our own family issues--kids, chores, personal relationships. What often happens is we are not patient, supportive, or tender with those people we care about the most. I remember my husband commenting one day that I wouldn't talk to a stranger in the manner I had just spoken to him. He was right. All too often it seems easier to be kind and more attentive to strangers than it is to those closest to us.

## *Laughter And Tears*

If we let it, this job of dealing with death could become overwhelmingly heavy. Our families and patients are distressed; their lives are changing dramatically. They are frightened, uncertain, depressed, and very sad.

We can't take their feelings and experience into

ourselves. We must find and experience joy, humor, and laughter - not at someone else's expense - but in the knowledge that it is healthy.

Laughter is a way of releasing tension, and sometimes it comes out in dark humor, inside jokes that only someone in our profession would find funny. Actually, we laugh not because it's all that funny, but as a release. Sometimes this makes us feel guilty: "Did I really say that? Did I really just laugh at that? OMG!" Dark humor and inside jokes are a part of any stressful profession. It isn't shared with outsiders, people who would not understand. This humor is not necessarily disrespectful (although it can be), but always needs to be seen for what it is—-a release of tension.

Humor and laughter are ways of releasing steam from the pressure cooker. (Where do you think the expression "letting off steam" comes from?) Laughter is a healthy way of decreasing tension, as is crying.

Tears are part of our job. Some situation or some happening will touch us on a personal level and tears will come. Acknowledge them, honor their sanctity, then wipe them off and move on. If you cry all the time it is a sign you are in the wrong job.

Occasional, situational tears show our humanity.

After I have had a tearful reaction with or about a patient I ask myself: "What did these tears mean? Where did they come from? Why?" Exploring the reason, taking the tears from an emotional to a mental level helps with the release of the tension. It puts the situation in perspective and allows us to move onto the next patient. Some of our most profound stories involve tears; our soul was touched and leaked out of our eyes.

## We Can't Fix Everything

We are in our patient and their family's lives for one reason: to help them have a meaningful, gentle dying experience. To do that, we support, guide, teach, and provide physical, emotional, and spiritual care. We are not there to change or judge the way a person has chosen to live their life. Yet so often we get into people's lives, see their struggling and dysfunction, and want to "fix" everything. Not our job! When we are guiding a family, if we find we're spending energy trying to "fix" a dysfunction outside of the dying process, we need to step back and remember the reason we're there. Also, if we are spending more energy to solve a problem that IS related to the dying process than the family involved, we need to remember that some battles can't be won. Continually trying to fight them isn't taking care of yourself. We offer guidance, knowledge, and opportunities. What people do with our offerings is up to them.

## We Don't Have All The Answers

Sometimes it is more helpful to listen to a person's story than to tell them how to solve their problems, even if you think you know the solutions. Sometimes just sitting there in silence is the best thing we can give. Yet we often create stress for ourselves because we can't fix problems, or have no idea how to help.

A large part of our responsibility to the families of our patients is education about end of life. For that we have answers. But for another part of our work, support and comfort, there are often no answers to the many questions asked. "Why me? Why my mother? What if the treatment had been different? How long does she have?"

There are no concrete answers to those questions (and we hear them asked all the time). We can only encourage the person asking to tell their story, to verbalize their thoughts and feelings while we quietly listen. A part of our job is to be good listeners.

Something to remember: Anytime you put a number on how long someone has to live you will probably be wrong and lose your credibility. The closest we can get is months, weeks, days or hours.

## *We Can't Carry the Pain*

Life is hard work. Working as a caregiver puts us into peoples lives at a time of crisis and turmoil. We see daily struggles, sadness, and pain of all kinds. In order for us to stay healthy and continue working we have to learn not to take on the struggles and challenges of others. It is so easy to get caught up in the lives of those for whom we are caring. Yet it is imperative that we remember that it is not our story, not our challenge, not our experience.

We cannot become emotionally involved in someone else's pain. Carrying someone else's challenges doesn't help them. We all have our own life situations to deal with, our own pain. Actually, by getting emotionally involved with our patient/family's struggles we create more stress for ourselves, thus making us less effective for them. We need to continually remind ourselves of our goal--to help a patient and their family have a gentle, peaceful dying experience. It is not our experience. It can be sad, traumatic, often dysfunctional, but it is not ours to carry. Do the best you can, offer the greatest assistance you have to give, then leave the situation at the patient's place of residence and move on.

## *Don't Take Negative Behavior Personally*

This is hard to do. Sick people can get downright cranky, as can their stressed families. As the caregiver you are often the easiest target. Anger at other family members, or even towards the patient, can get directed at the caregiver because it is safer than confronting the person with whom they are really upset. That behavior is not about you. It is in your best interest to not take the outbursts or comments personally. That said, there is no reason to withstand insults, abusive language, untruths, or being yelled at.

You can calmly (operative word is calmly) say "This is unacceptable. If you continue I will leave."

## Find Someone To Talk To

As a caregiver working with end of life, it is important to not keep all the tragedy, sadness, and intensity of other peoples' lives inside your life--- yet confidentiality dictates you keep quiet. This is an unhealthy paradox. Find someone with whom to share, who understands your work environment, who will not necessarily have answers but will listen to you talk. A weekly get together with other caregivers is a great way to unwind. A little food, a beverage, a relaxing atmosphere, and a lot of sharing can greatly reduce the daily tensions of our high stress job.

Needing to talk, and be listened to, is not the sign of weakness that we tend to think it is. It is the reality of our jobs. We see, interact with, and are expected to have answers for issues that most human beings choose not to think about, let alone experience. We interact on a daily basis with difficult, challenging, and unusual situations.

We are not weak. We are strong. And one of the ways to stay strong is to find someone who will appreciate your experiences, someone to talk to.

After a particularly intense experience it is beneficial to debrief immediately. My "in the field" protocol was for nurses, social workers, nurse's aides and chaplains to call me immediately following any situation that may have upset them. They were to tell me right away their "story", to recount what had happened in all its often grizzly detail. This quick release prevents the images from "sticking" to us. It gives us the assurance we are not alone, that we are safe.

If your agency does not offer that immediate phone call opportunity, find someone you can trust to be your touchstone. Set this up ahead of time, before you need to make the phone call. No answers are needed, no judgements, just a listening ear. This debriefing is a step by step recounting of the events. The retelling releases pent up intensities, emotions, uncertainties, and sometimes fears and horrors. You are releasing, letting go, so you can continue on. Again, very important to remember, this is not a sign of weakness, it is good mental health.

# Life's Appreciation

Dying is not a medical event. It is a social, communal experience. It isn't our medical expertise that will help us be effective, it is our social skills, our listening skills, and our knowledge of the dying process and our end of life skills that are valuable.

Working in end of life is like being a salmon, you're always swimming against the current. As caregivers, our skills are contrary to much of what we have been medically taught. It is important to recognize that people may not understand the care we are providing. They may question our approach. We need to be confident in our knowledge, our skills, and within ourselves. If we have self-confidence we can go home at the end of the day and feel good about the special interactions we have had.

Working with end of life reminds us of the precariousness of life. It shows us the gift we have in just being able to get out of bed in the morning. The gift of being able to reach out to others with a helping hand. Gratitude and appreciation for the life we have is the gift our patients and families give us.

It can be fulfilling to work in a job that brings direction and meaning into the lives of others. BUT in order to do that job effectively and continuously we must keep our own body and mind healthy and balanced. We need a sense of fulfillment, peace of mind in our being, and joy in our life. Here is some daily food for thought, goals and self evaluation questions for assessing the quality of each day. I use them before I go to sleep at night as a gentle reminder of how I want to live my life.

- What was good about today?
- Did I experience love, joy, and fulfillment?
- What did I learn?
- Were my interactions with others genuine and satisfying?
- What changes do I want to make if I want my answers to the above to be different?
- Was what I did today worth trading a day of my life for?

*I work with dying people, all of my patients die.*
*I see grief and sadness and anger and depression.*
*Most is an individual's internal anguish needing to be brought out, to be worked out.*
*Nowhere is it written that life will always be the way we'd like it to be.*
*Dying presents us with perhaps the greatest opportunity for growth we have ever had.*
*This struggle is part of life; it is a learning process--*
*Learning to live, learning to die*
*That is what physical life is all about.*
*There is no pain for me here.*
*Today I walked into a hospital room.*
*My patient/friend was strapped in a wheel chair, facing a blank wall, his back turned to a blaring TV and the door.*
*His body heavy and uncomfortable falling limply over the side of the chair.*
*His arm blue from hanging too long a time at his side.*
*Unable to talk because of a brain tumor,*
*Unable to maneuver his body,*
*He was trapped by someone else's hurriedness.*
*Poop on his hands, from poop in his pants,*
*He took my hand in his and kissed it--*
*A thank you for getting him back into bed*
*And my heart cried.*
*Here lies my pain!*
*The indignities that need not be in life for lessons to be learned.*
*The indignities imposed upon a human being by another human being.*
*Herein lies my pain!*

— Barbara Karnes, RN

## *Summary*

Working with end of life is not like most of the work we have been trained to do. We are trained to help people get better, not to die.

Everything we do is because it meets a need within ourselves. Examine why you are doing end of life work.

It isn't just our knowledge that we bring to the lives of the people we touch. We bring our belief system, our fears, our guilt, our childhood experiences: the very foundation our personality is built upon. Because of this we need to examine our beliefs and experiences carefully.

We will grieve the loss of our patient whether we recognize it or not. To address that grief we can create a closure ritual.

Areas to balance: eating, sleep, play, family, and work. A lot of us sacrifice sleep and play for work while over compensating in the eating department.

Humor and laughter can be letting the steam out of the pressure cooker.

Acknowledge your tears and honor their sanctity, then wipe them off and continue your work. If you cry all the time it is a sign you are in the wrong job. Occasional tears show our humanity.

It is not our job to "fix" all the dysfunction a family has spent a lifetime creating.

If we are spending more energy to solve a problem that is related to the dying process than the family involved, we need to remember that some battles can't be won.

Sometimes it is more helpful to listen to someone's story than to tell them how to solve their problems.

By getting emotionally involved with our patient/family's struggles we create more stress for ourselves, thus making us less effective for them.

It is in our best interest to not take negative outbursts or comments personally.

There is no reason to withstand insults, abusive language, untruths, or being yelled at. We can calmly say "This is unacceptable. If you continue I will leave."

When working with end of life situations it is important to keep all the tragedy, sadness, and intensity of other peoples' lives at the office and not carry them home with us.

Find someone with whom to share your experiences, feelings and ideas.

The debriefing of intense experiences is imperative to staying healthy.

It isn't necessarily our medical knowledge that will help us be effective. It is our social, listening, and end of life skills that are valuable.

We need a sense of fulfillment, peace of mind in our being, and joy in our life.

# NEW RULES
## for end of life care

## Informative & Engaging DVD Kit

**Consistent Family Education**
for nurses and social workers to watch with families.

**Continuing Education**
for staff & volunteer inservice, training and orientation.

**Marketing & Community Outreach**
for acquiring referrals, promoting services, community education and growing your business.

Winner of Multiple International Awards

BARBARA KARNES RN

**AWARD WINNING**
end of life educator and hospice pioneer

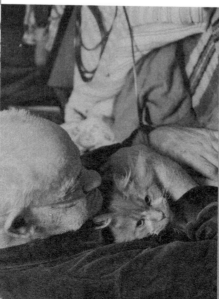

Caring for someone as they approach the end of their life is not the same as caring for a person who is going to get better. Unfortunately, most people don't know this. "New Rules For End of Life Care" is an educational kit to be read and viewed at the patient's home, in a nursing facility, hospice/palliative care or hospital.

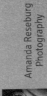
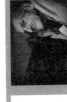
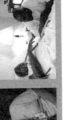
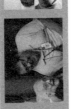
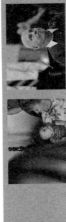

Amanda Reseburg Photography

cost: $29 per kit + shipping

## Contents

### DVD: New Rules
Important information on end of life care that addresses behavior changes as they pertain to food, sleep and pain management.

### Blue Booklet: Gone From My Sight
Detailed information on what you should expect to see in the months, weeks, days and hours approaching death from old age or disease.

### Pink Booklet: The Eleventh Hour
A caring guideline for the hours to minutes before death.

to place an order or view the DVD trailer, please visit www.bkbooks.com or call 360-828-7132
Barbara Karnes Books, Inc.   PO Box 822139  Vancouver, WA 98682

# Barbara Karnes Books, Inc. ORDER FORM  www.bkbooks.com - bkbooks@bkbooks.com

Please write total quantity of booklets next to translation.
Use reverse side for books, compilations, DVD's, grand total for order, and your shipping information.

**Gone From My Sight**  English____ Spanish____ French____ Russian____ Italian____
Korean____ Vietnamese____ Japanese____

**The Eleventh Hour**  English____ Spanish____
**A Time To Live**  English____ Spanish____
**My Friend, I Care**  English____ Spanish____ French____
**How Do I Know You?**  English____

**The Tree of Life & Family Tree** Children's coloring/Adult Art Therapy)  English____
**I Am Standing Upon The Seashore** (Children's coloring/Adult Art Therapy) English____

### Pricing & Discounts for booklets

|  |  |
|---|---|
| 1 - 99 | $2.00 per copy |
| 100 - 249 | $1.80 per copy |
| 250 - 499 | $1.70 per copy |
| 500 - 999 | $1.60 per copy |

Please call 360-828-7132 for discounts on orders of 1000 or more copies.

Total number of copies (from booklets above) Quantity # _____

Price per copy (from chart on right) $ _____

7% KS Tax (Kansas customers only) $ _____

8.4% WA Tax (Washington customers only) $ _____

Postage & Handling (from chart on right) $ _____

**Total $ _____**

### Postage & Handling

|  |  |
|---|---|
| 1 copy | $2.00 |
| 2 copies | $3.00 |
| 3 - 10 copies | $4.00 |
| 11 - 25 copies | $5.00 |
| 26 - 50 copies | $7.00 |
| 51 - 100 copies | $9.00 |
| 101 - 250 copies | $17.00 |
| 251 - 350 copies | $22.00 |
| 351 - 500 copies | $27.00 |

Booklet orders may be combined to achieve a discount.
Pricing includes any combination of booklets. All available languages are listed to the right of the booklet title.
Postage may be adjusted for rate increases. Please visit www.bkbooks.com for discounts and postage rates not listed, secure credit card orders, new materials and eBooks.
Custom cover branding now available. Please call for more information.

~Please use reverse side for more materials and address information~
Custom cover branding now available! Call for information.

Name / Agency _____

Contact _____

PO# _____

Address _____

City _____

State _____ Zip _____

Phone _____ Fax _____

E-Mail _____

## New Rules For End of Life Care Kit
New Rules DVD plus two booklets;
Gone From My Sight and The Eleventh Hour.
*Multi - Award Winner!*

Quantity # _____
$29.00 per kit $ _____
Postage $4.00 per kit $ _____

*Call for correct postage and discounts on multiple kits.*

Total $ _____

## Knowledge Reduces Fear
An easy to read printed collection of
Barbara's blog articles and comments.

Volume 1 - Quantity # _____
$5.00 per copy $ _____
Postage $3.00 per copy $ _____

*Call for correct postage on multiple copies.*

Total $ _____

## The Final Act of Living - *Reflections of a Longtime Hospice Nurse*
Insights and perceptions from years of working with people during their final act of living.
259 page book. English only.

Quantity # _____
$15 per copy $ _____
Postage $4.00 per copy $ _____

Total $ _____

*Call for correct postage and discounts on multiple copies*

## Training DVD's (Postage included in price for the following DVD's)

Dynamics of Dying (2 DVD set) *$300.00 ea*   Qty # _____ Total $ _____

Grief: Exploring The Process (1 DVD) *$100.00 ea*   Qty # _____ Total $ _____

Total for above materials *(including postage)* $ _____

Booklet order total *(including postage)* from other side $ _____

**GRAND TOTAL FOR ORDER** $ _____

## MAIL TO:
**Barbara Karnes Books, Inc.**
Po Box 822139
Vancouver, WA 98682

Phone (9-4 pm PST) 360-828-7132
Fax 360-828-7142
**www.bkbooks.com**